Willow Wonders
Why do I Worry?

Written by
Wynne & Kristin Beckstrom Radcliffe, MSW, LCSW
Illustrated by Jeremy Provost

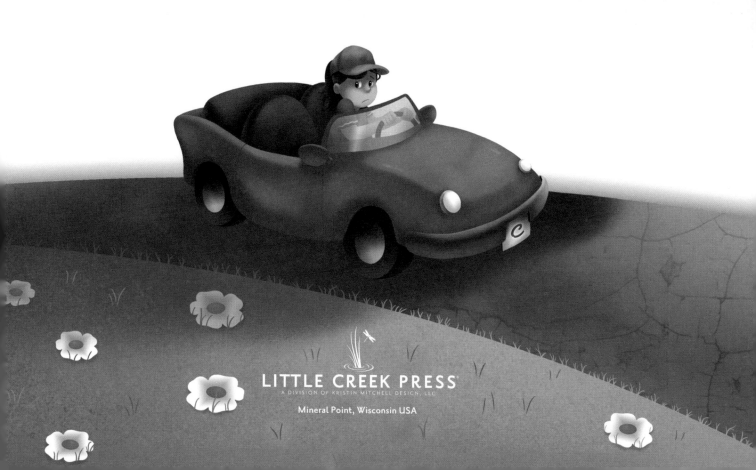

LITTLE CREEK PRESS
A DIVISION OF KRISTIN MITCHELL DESIGN, LLC

Mineral Point, Wisconsin USA

Little Creek Press®
A Division of Kristin Mitchell Design, LLC
5341 Sunny Ridge Road
Mineral Point, Wisconsin 53565

Illustrator: Jeremy Provost
Editor: Bob Wake and Carrie Stidwell O'Bogle
Book Design and Project Coordination: Little Creek Press

Limited First Edition
October 2013

Printed in Wisconsin, United States of America.

For more information or to order books:
www.littlecreekpress.com

Library of Congress Control Number: 2013947338

ISBN-10: 0989643123
ISBN-13: 978-0-9896431-2-2

Dedication

To my favorite veteran,
my Sugar Plum and Rockstar.

~ KBR

To Peyton and Ayanna for taking me
as I am and to my family who has
helped me through all of this.

~ WVR

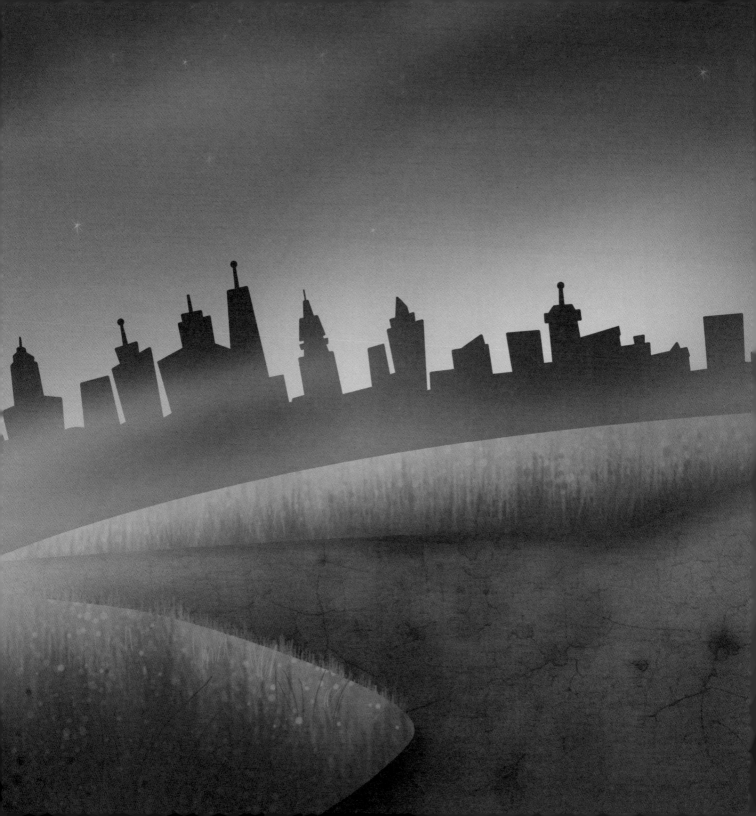

What is OCD?
A note to Parents and Teachers

In short, obsessive compulsive disorder (OCD) is an anxiety disorder in which people have unwanted and repeated thoughts, feelings, ideas, sensations (obsessions) or behaviors that make them feel driven to do something. The obsessions can be related to contamination, loss of control, harm to self or others, perfectionism, religious or moral obsessions, or superstitious ideas about numbers or colors. Common compulsions include washing or cleaning, checking, repeating, hoarding or collecting, mental compulsions (e.g. counting while performing a task) or putting things in order or arranging them until it feels just right.

OCD can exist on its own or can be co-morbid (also exist) with other disorders. It is not a disorder that can fit in a box; and it is not just regular worries about every day situations. When a person is truly distressed, the obsessions and/or compulsions take more than an hour a day, and the obsessions/compulsions interfere with normal activities. Further attention must be paid and support initiated.

Willow Wonders is designed to educate the unfamiliar and begin a discussion, from the unique perspective of a child. We desperately want people to better understand the challenges of being a kid who worries and encourage respect and compassion. While the message here is positive, this is a serious topic and one, we believe, that needs more understanding and attention. We have the confidence that anyone who reads *Willow Wonders* will gain faith in a child's ability to grow. We want to encourage children and their families who deal with anxiety and OCD on a daily basis to recognize that the process of growth and adjustment are continuous. The map and coping strategies of the seven year old are not the same as the growing tween or adolescent.

Please let this book start discussions, point people in the directions of hope and healing. Find what works best for your student, your family. Let our maps be a place of beginning.

Warmly,
Wynne Radcliffe
Kristin Beckstrom Radcliffe, MSW, LCSW

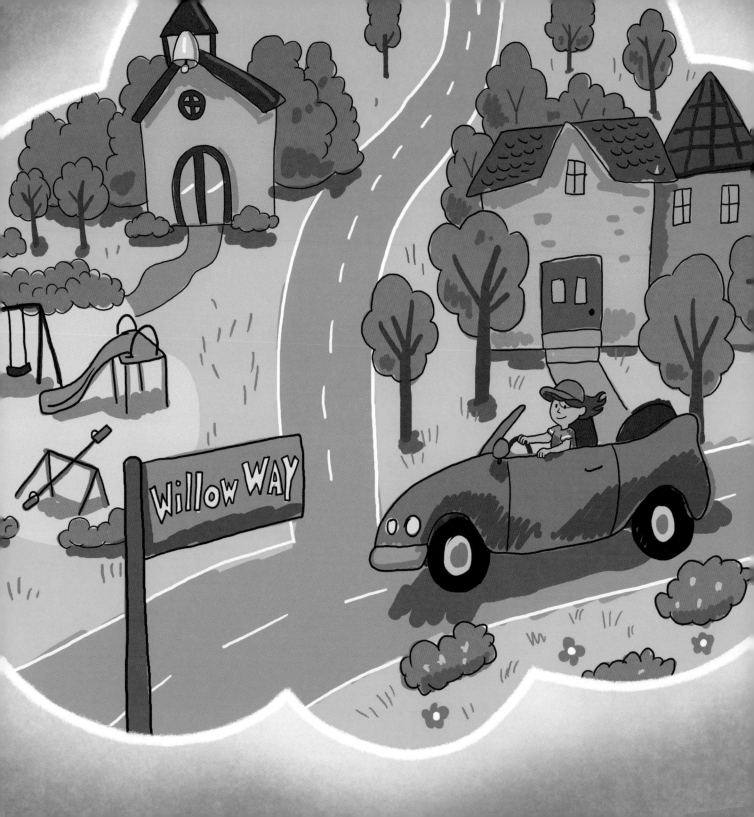

My name is Willow and sometimes I worry.
My thoughts are a street named Willow Way.
I like to imagine myself driving a
pink car named Charlotte.

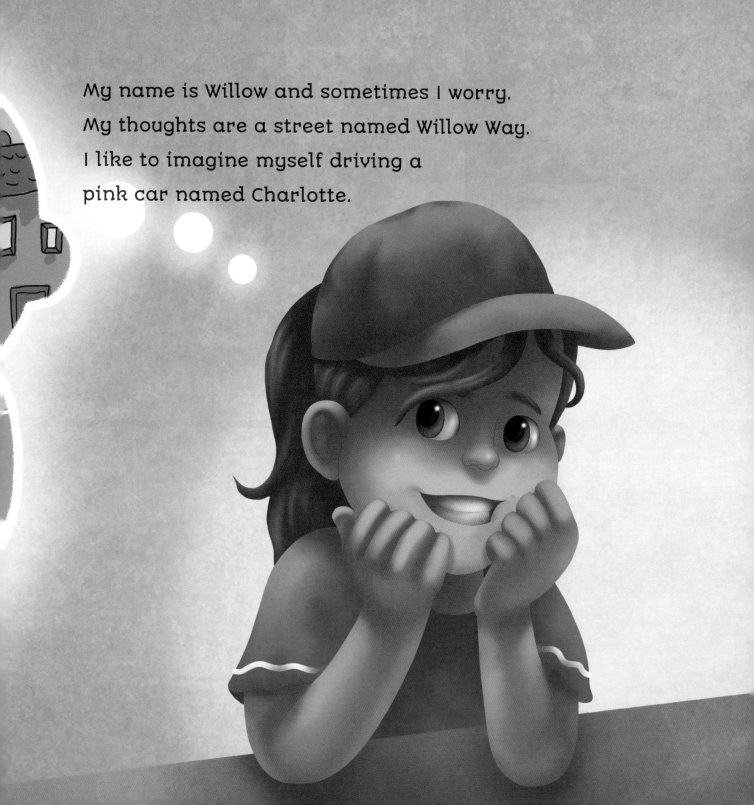

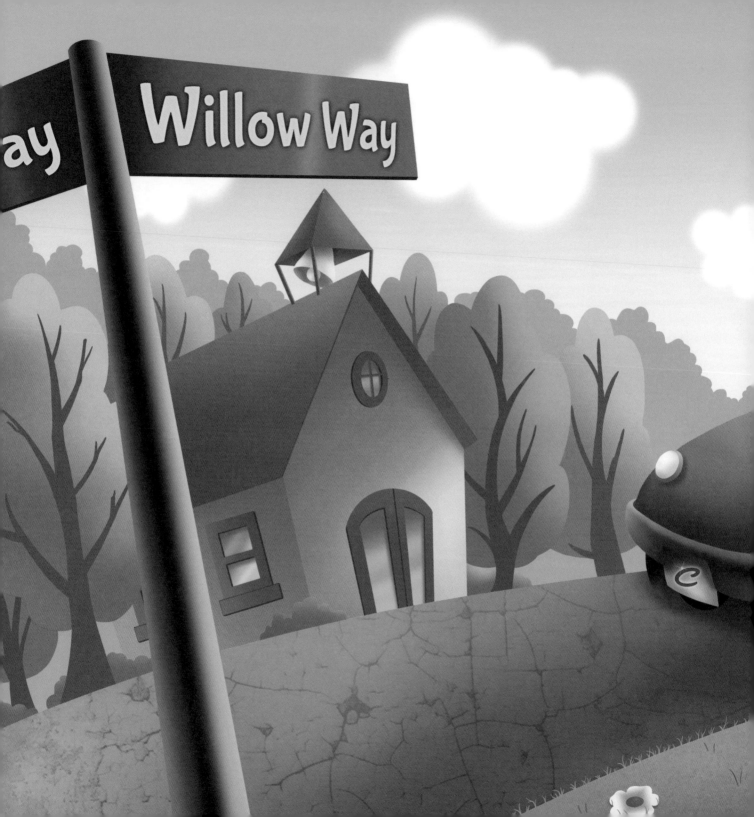

Some days I have a perfect map in my head.
Willow Way is clear of traffic and the sun
is shining as I drive to school.
I feel calm and happy.

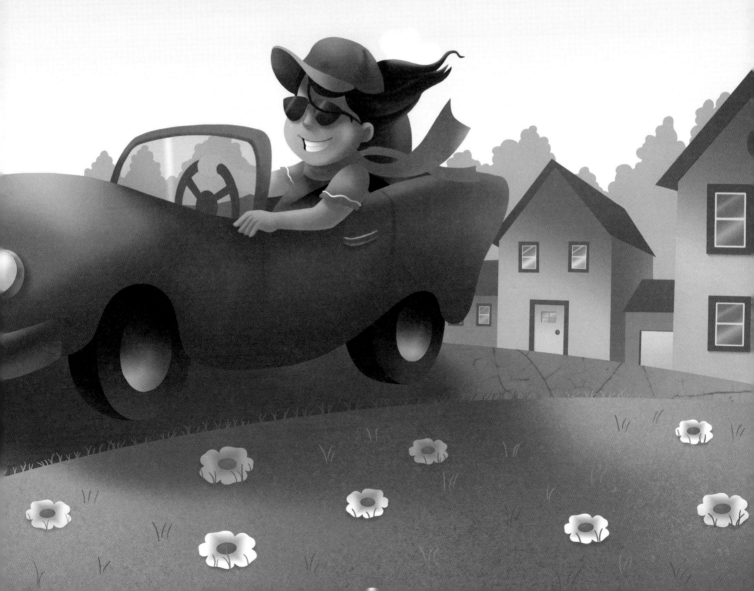

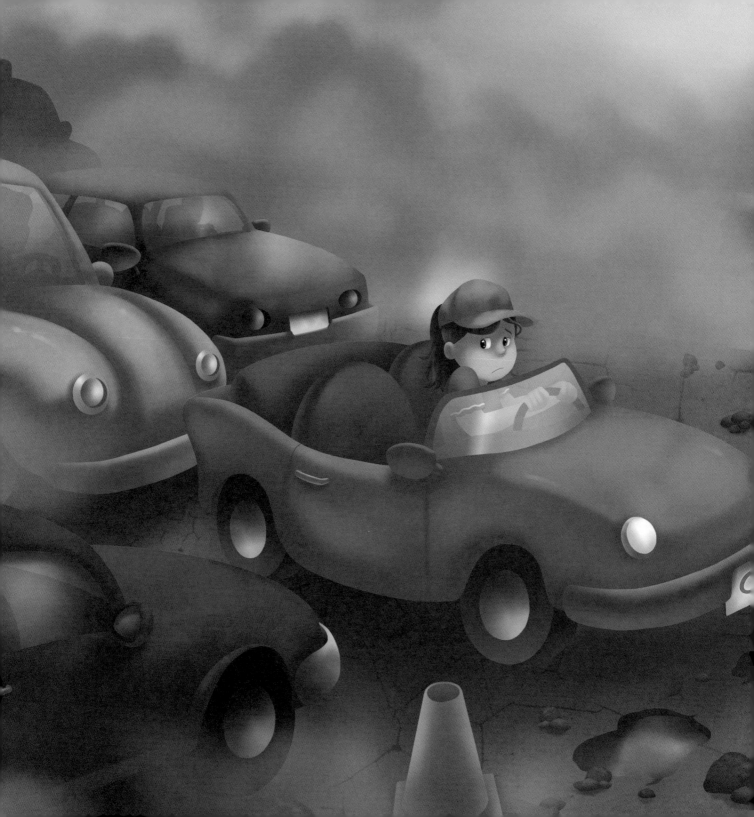

On other days, my map is a mess. Willow Way is
bumpy and filled with angry red cars honking.
My messed-up map worries me. Where am I going?
Will I get there? Why do I worry?

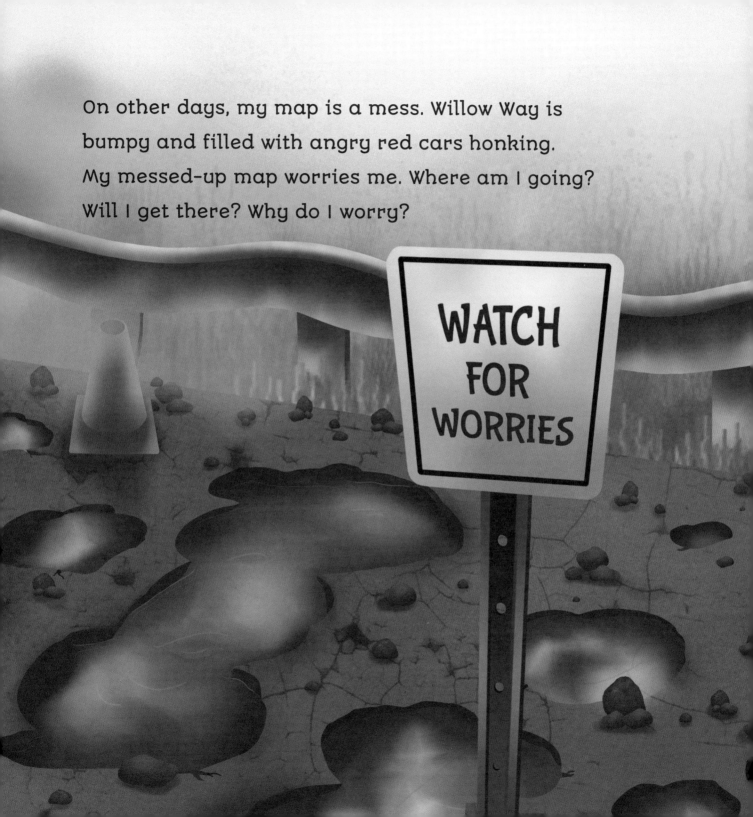

WATCH
FOR
WORRIES

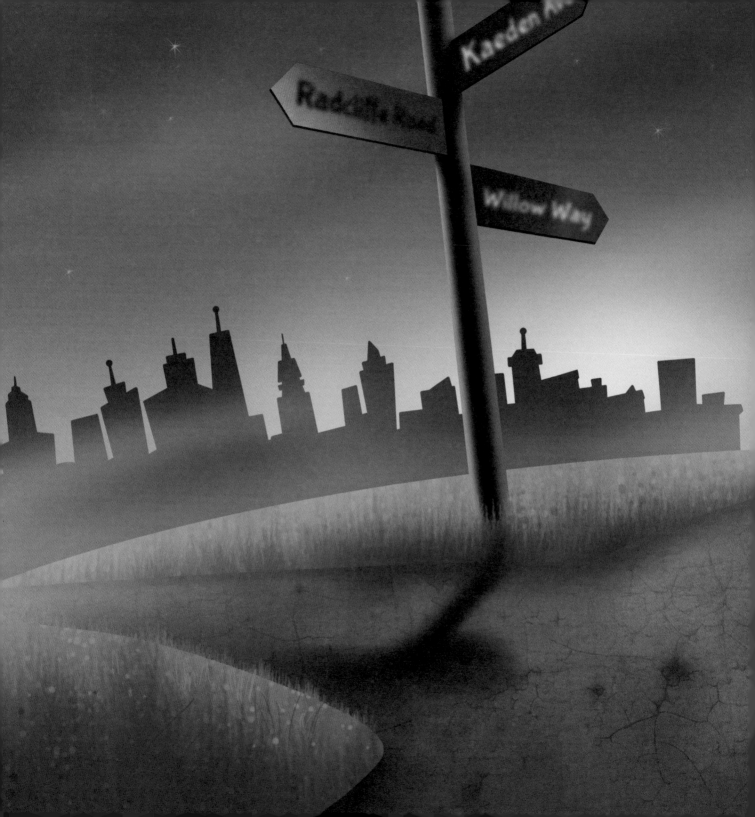

I ask mom and dad, "Do your maps
ever get jammed up and crazy?"
"Sure," they say. "When the road signs
are hard to read and we lose our way."

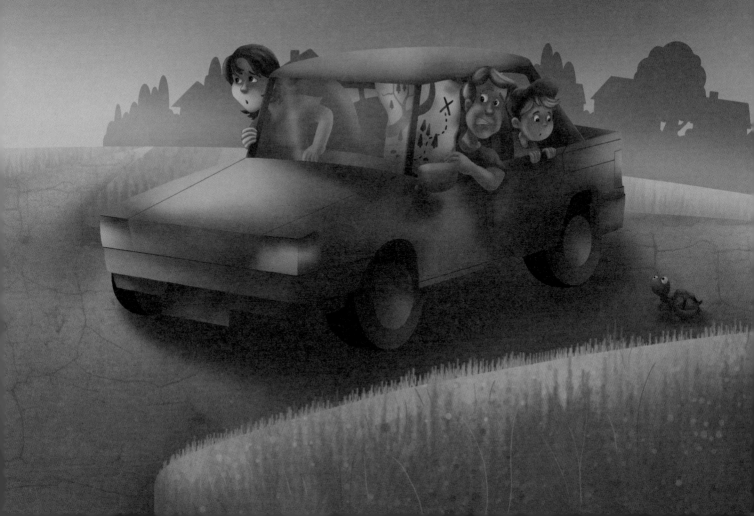

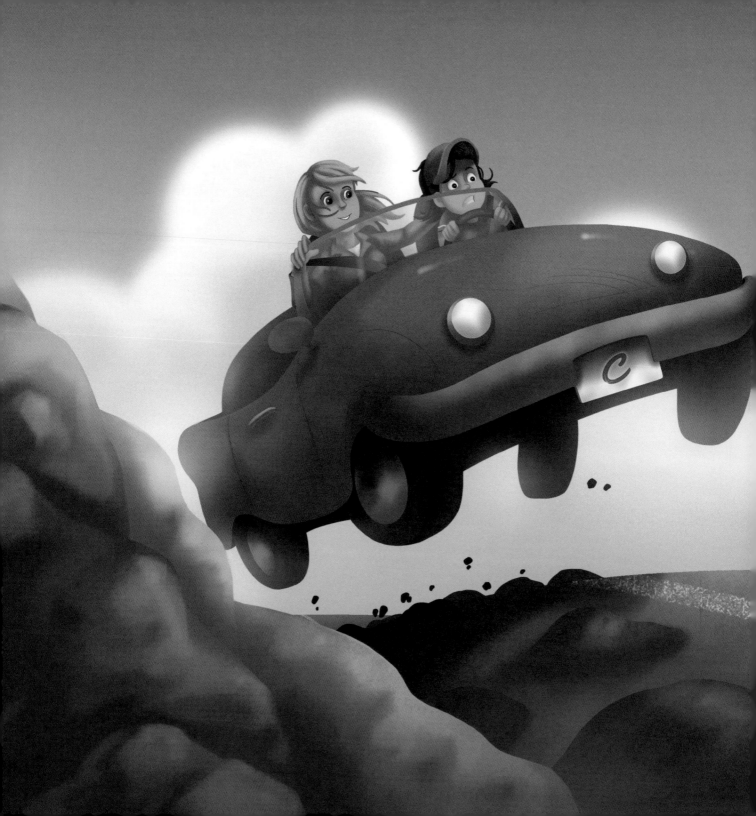

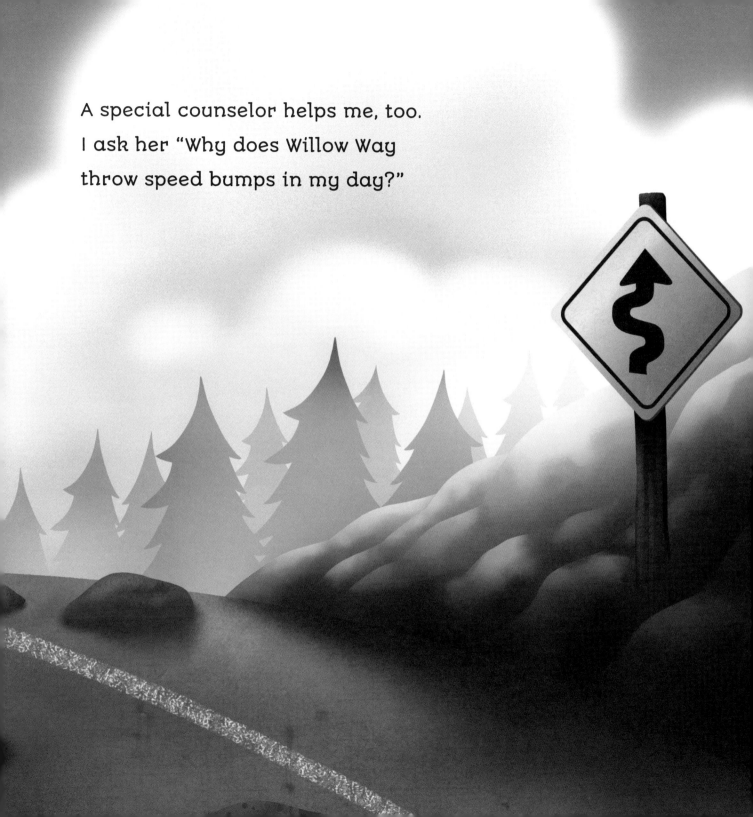

A special counselor helps me, too.
I ask her "Why does Willow Way
throw speed bumps in my day?"

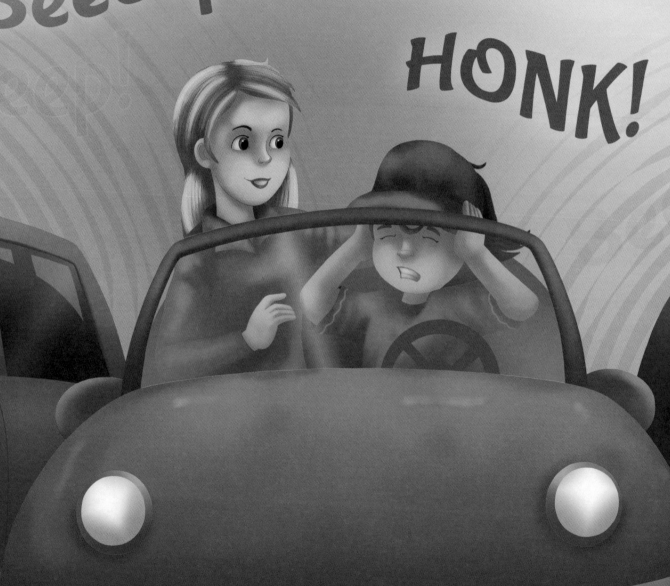

She says, "Sometimes a worry is like a loud car alarm that won't stop. If you can turn down your alarm, you can calm down your map."

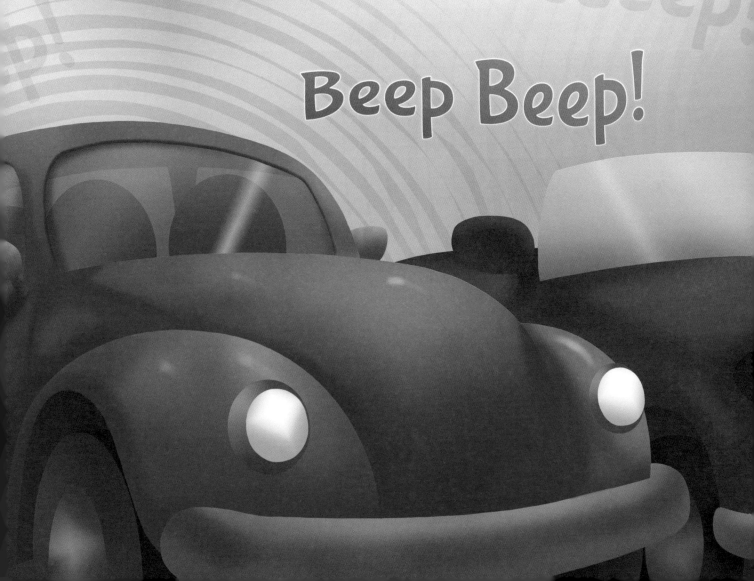

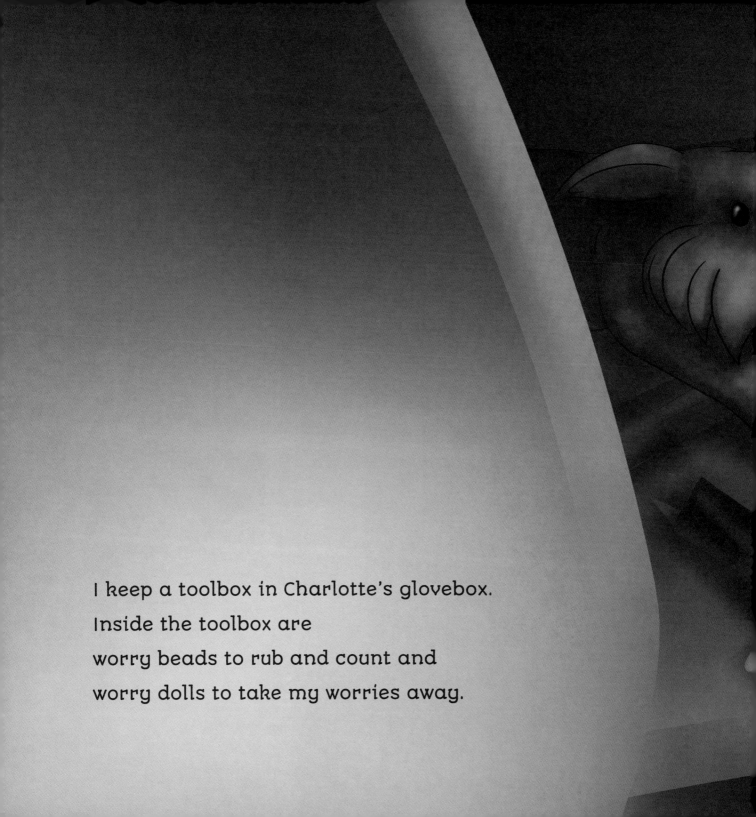

I keep a toolbox in Charlotte's glovebox.
Inside the toolbox are
worry beads to rub and count and
worry dolls to take my worries away.

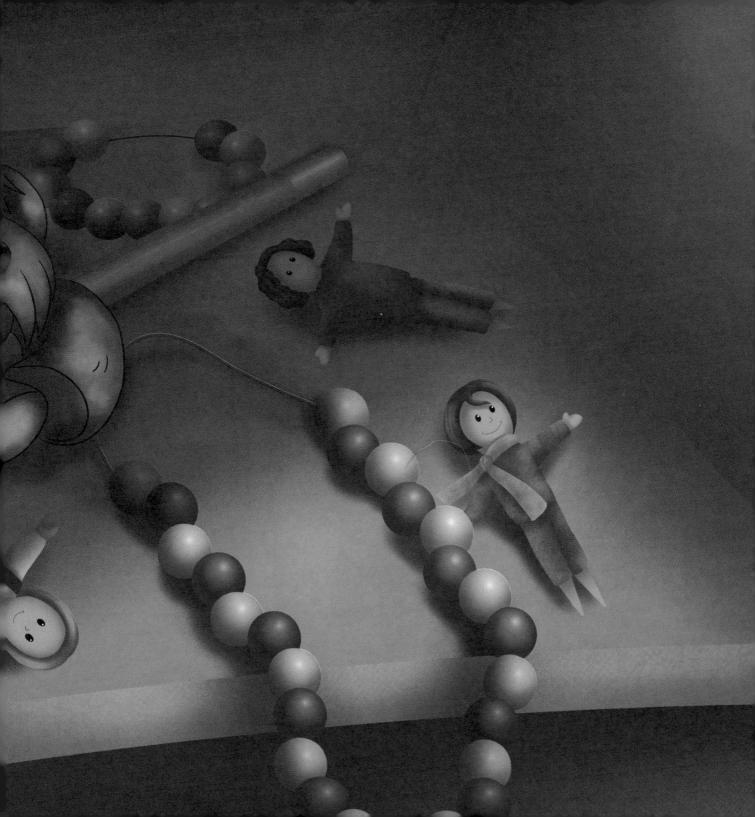

I can turn down the alarms by using
the tools in my toolbox.
I can repair the road by filling the potholes.
I can clear the traffic to stop the honking.

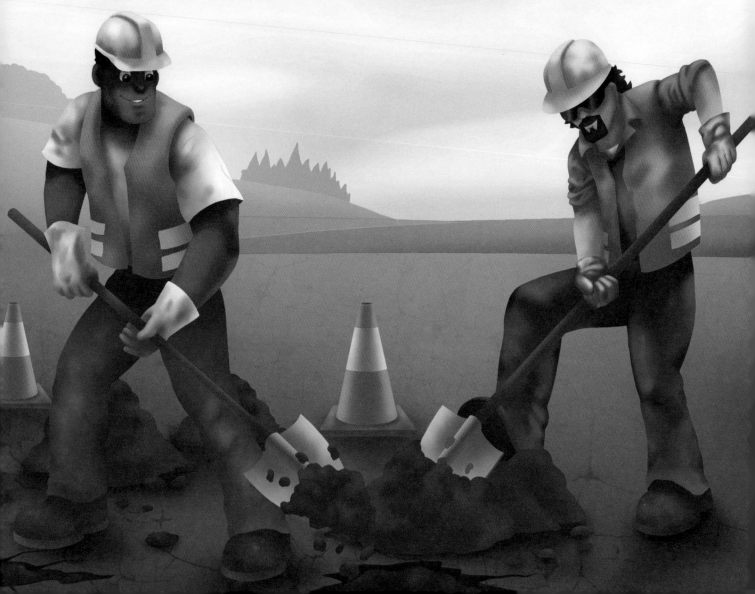

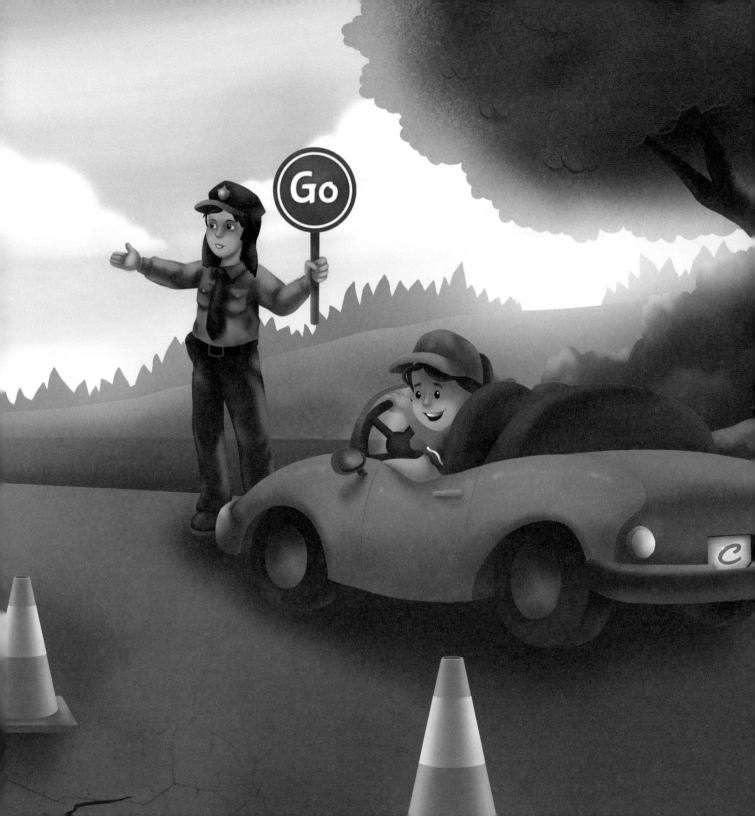

Then Charlotte and I can
continue on Willow Way.

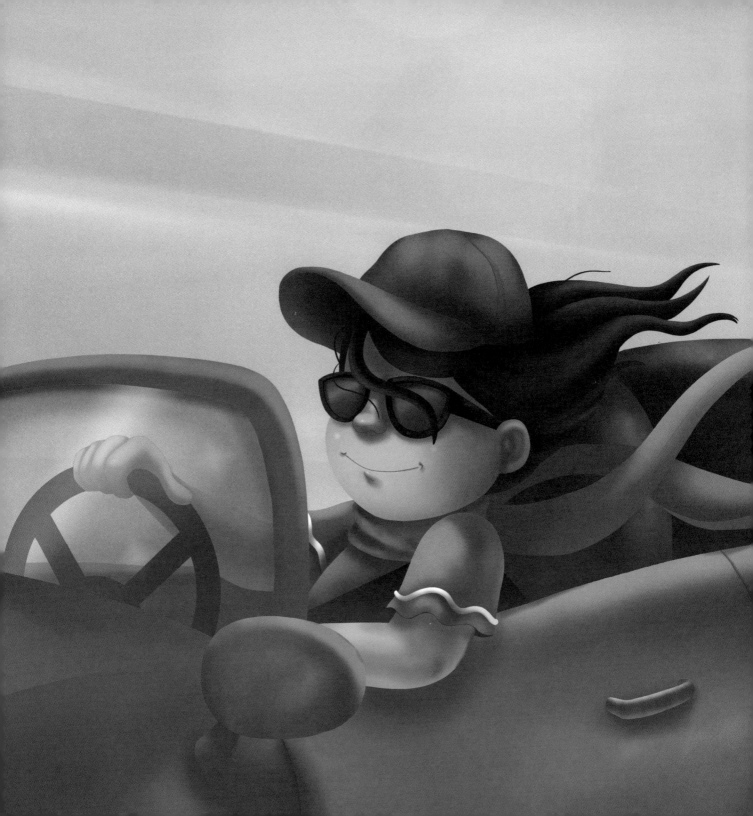

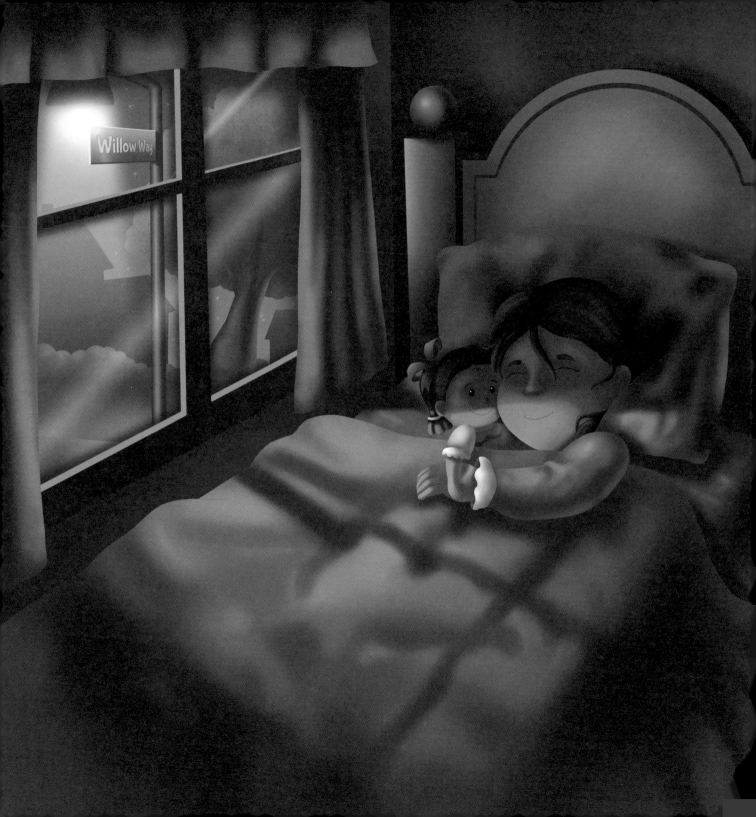

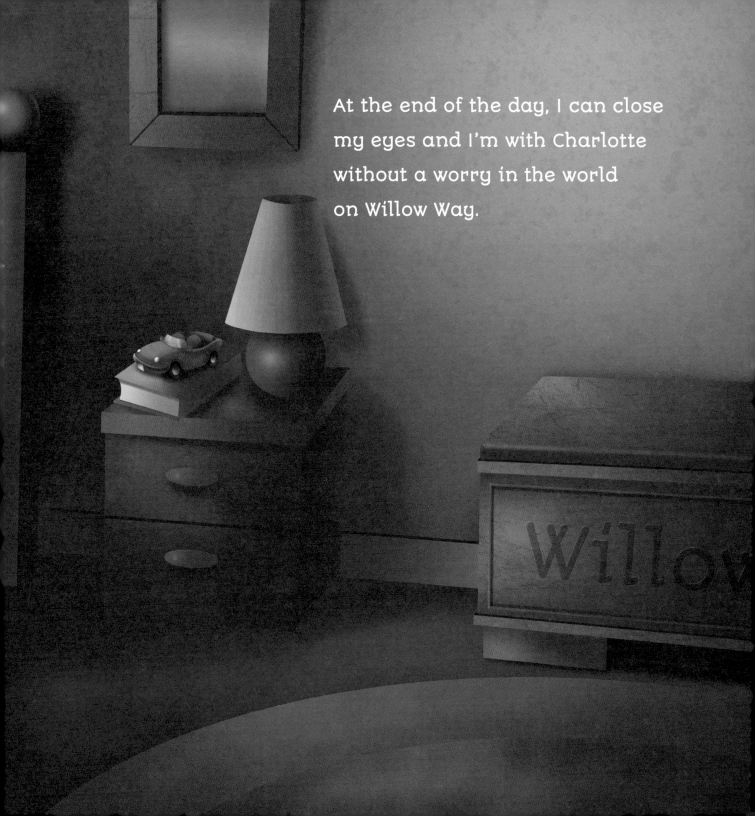

At the end of the day, I can close my eyes and I'm with Charlotte without a worry in the world on Willow Way.

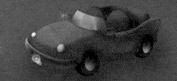

The End

ABOUT THE AUTHORS

Wynne

Wynne is an eleven-year-old sixth grader who deals with OCD and worry every day. She was lucky to be a military kid, living in Alabama, Germany and Illinois until her dad retired. She is a devoted and loyal big sister to her brother Kaeden, a second grader. She adores TaeKwonDo, playing school, and all things Harry Potter.

Kristin

Kristin is a mom and social worker, currently in private practice. She

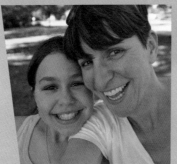

has worked in a variety of social services settings in her career, including schools, military facilities and child protection agencies. She discovered running at 35 and currently loves her turtle paced triathlons. Kristin fiercely loves her own kiddos and her husband, but also loves sharing her gifts with countless others.

Jeremy Provost

Jeremy Provost was born in Oconomowoc, a small lake country town in Wisconsin. As a child Jeremy was introduced to Bill Watterson's Calvin and Hobbes, which instantly grounded his desire to become a comic illustrator. After years of being told he couldn't draw in class, Jeremy decided to become a student at Indiana Wesleyan University. While enrolled Jeremy taught under children's illustrtrator Ron Mazellan. Ron's mentorship and guidance was very influential in Jeremy's own shift of passion toward children's illustra-

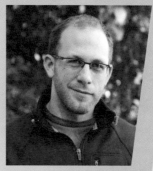

tion. Jeremy graduated IWU in the summer of 2008 with an illustration degree, and ventured back home.

Jeremy was eventually contacted by Little Creek Press, a small publishing company in his home state. Through Little Creek Press, Jeremy received the opportunity to complete his first Children's book, "Jumpin' Jackie, The Cow That Jumped Over The Moon."

Jeremy has since then worked on various projects, and now spends his days as an active children's illustrator. His greatest desire is to spark imagination to a younger audience, just as "Calvin and Hobbes" sparked his own as a child.

Resources

The Anxiety and Depression Association of America

www.adaa.org

The ADAA is a leader in education, training and research. They are a non-profit organization that provides information and support for patients, their families and professionals. They are dedicated to increasing awareness and improving the diagnosis, treatment and cure of anxiety disorders in children and adults.

The International OCD Foundation

www.ocdfoundation.org

The International OCD foundation is an international non-profit organization made up of people with OCD and related disorders, their families, friends, and professionals who work with them. They aim to educate the public and improve the quality of treatement, support research, improve access to resources and advocate and lobby for the OCD community.

The National Alliance on Mental Illness

www.nami.org

NAMI is the nation's largest non-profit, grassroots mental health education, advocacy and support organization dedicated to building better lives for those affected by mental illness. Local and state chapters are present and active throughout the country.

The American Psychiatric Association

www.apa.org

The APA is the organization behind the development of the Diagnostic and Statistical Manual for Mental Disorders (DSM). In the Spring of 2013, an updated DSM-5 was released. While they are responsible for the manual by which many diagnoses are made, they are also at the forefront of ongoing research into mental illnesses.

Helpful Books

"What to do when your brain gets stuck" Dawn Huebner, PhD

"What to do when you worry too much" Dawn Huebner, PhD

"Wilma Jean the Worry Machine" Julia Cook

"Wilma Jean the Worry Machine
- Activity and Idea Book" Julia Cook

"Take Control of OCD – The Ultimate Guide
for Kids with OCD" Bonnie Zucker, PsyD

"Anxiety-Free Kids: An Interactive Guide
for Parents and Children" Bonnie Zucker, PsyD

"Freeing your child from anxiety: Powerful
practical solutions to overcome your child's
fears, worries and phobias" Tamar Chansky

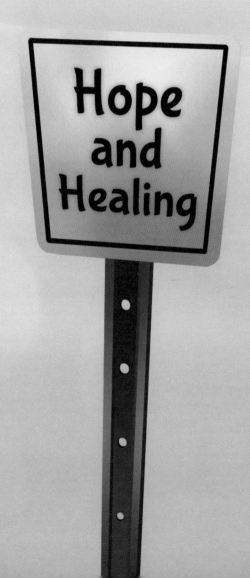

Thank you!